Introduction

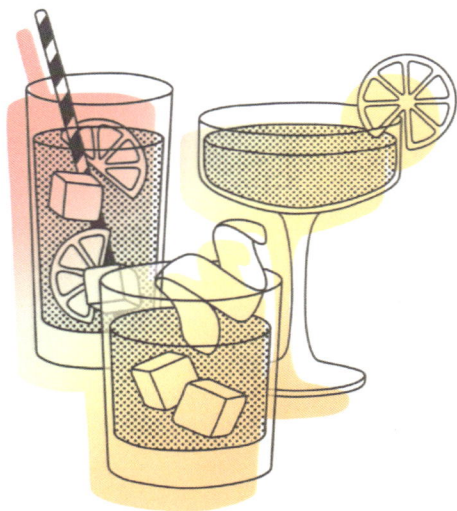

We know that getting enough fluid in each day to support your body's needs can be a challenge. However, we believe hydration doesn't have to be boring and a 'nice drink' doesn't need to involve alcohol.

We created this book for anyone that is looking for some fun new ways to enjoy electrolytes, especially those who live with Orthostatic Intolerance (OI), Postural Orthostatic Tachycardia Syndrome (POTS) or Dysautonomia, as electrolytes can be very beneficial for those living with these conditions.

We have tried, tested and collated recipes to help you spice up the way you get your electrolytes in.

This book contains recipes for:

Reasons these recipes might be for you

You may be needing some holiday season inspiration and our electrolyte mocktail recipes aim to help hydrate, manage symptoms and not miss out on a fun and tasty drink. Alternatively, you might not have OI, POTS or Dysautonomia and just want to enjoy a good non-alcoholic beverage for the summer.

You may want some inspiration on some fun summer sweets that also help with getting in electrolytes in the process - snack and hydration in one, what more could you ask for?

You may be sick of, or unable to tolerate electrolyte products but want a way you can make it at home to suit those flavour and texture preferences, that electrolyte brands just don't hit.

You may be struggling with the heat in summer and need a way to both cool down and replenish the electrolytes you lose through sweat.

Why Electrolytes?

Electrolytes help to increase our sodium and fluid intake simultaneously to boost blood volume which helps to reduce OI and POTS symptoms. They help those with OI, POTS and Dysautonomia better retain fluid that their kidneys would otherwise choose to excrete due to blood pooling.

Electrolytes can also give water a more pleasant flavour which can help some people drink enough.

Check out a video from our Active Health Clinic (AHC) dietitian, Mel to learn more about why electrolytes can be helpful by scanning the QR code below:

Getting enough fluid and electrolytes in is especially important in summer for a number of reasons:

1. The heat dilates (expands) blood vessels. Imagine your blood vessels as a garden hose spraying water in a constant and strong stream. Now imagine all of a sudden it doubles in diameter - although the amount of water going in hasn't changed, the volume the water needs to fill has, therefore, the strong stream is lost and water trickles out of the hose. For anyone, this means we need to drink more and retain more fluid across the day in summer but this is especially important in those with OI, POTS and Dysautonomia as this may trigger symptoms.

Scan the below QR code for a video from our AHC dietitian, Mel to learn more:

2. We sweat more when it is hot. We also lose fluid and salt through our sweat. Therefore, we need to replenish what we lose throughout the day whether it be from just braving the heat or doing some movement and getting hot and sweaty. Electrolytes help with both fluid and salt loss.

3. We may need to cool down. Drinking (or in the case of this book, also snacking on) ice cold electrolytes can be a way to remain cool and help regulate temperature.

4. Help combat nausea. Firstly, sips of an ice cold fluid help distract the nervous system from the sensation of nausea. For those with OI, POTS and Dysautonomia, staying adequately hydrated can assist with reducing lack of blood flow to the gastrointestinal system and reduce nausea.

What Electrolytes should I use?

You might be thinking "There's so many electrolyte brands out there, how do I know which electrolytes to use?" and also "What is best, homemade or store bought electrolyte drinks?".

First of all, we have found there is no one "perfect" electrolyte drink as everyone's "perfect" is different. Some may prioritise taste, texture, cost/amount of sodium per serve, or intolerances/sensitivities etc.... the possibilities are endless.

The dietetics team at AHC have created a free "Electrolyte Comparison Document" (ECD) to help you to compare loads of electrolyte brands for your specific preferences and needs! We update this document at least yearly to keep up to date with changes in prices, new brands and more.

To access this document please scan the QR code below. This will take you to a webpage to fill out the details required. You will then be sent an email with a copy of the ECD and a video from AHC Dietitians explaining how to use it. Sending the ECD this way will allow us to send you the updated version in a more time effective way in the future.

If you have any feedback or specific questions regarding electrolytes please reach out to the team at:

- admin@activehealthclinic.com.au
- or message us through our Facebook (Active Health Clinic) or Instagram (@activehealthclinic_au)

What Electrolytes should I use?

Throughout the recipes in this book we have used a variety of different electrolyte brands and types to show you that you can get the desired effect with different electrolytes.
You can use and experiment with whatever electrolyte brands you prefer or have on hand.

However, we have chosen certain electrolytes for their flavour and texture profiles. These products are also the ones that AHC dietitians recommend to patients the most, as their clinical uses, as well as their sensory profiles, we believe, are the most widely applicable for those with OI, POTS and Dysautonomia. We sell all three brands of electrolytes used for recipes in our AHC shop as one of our core values is improving access to vital supports for people with invisible illnesses.

We are aiming to grow our store to be a one stop shop for all your invisible illness needs - so watch this space.

Speaking of accessibility, we've got a surprise gift for you!

A one off 10% discount code for electrolytes on the shop if you are wanting to try any of the brands used in this book (excludes 12 pack boxes of pH1500).

Head to our shop through scanning the QR code below and use code "recipe10" at the checkout:

Electrolytes used in our recipes

- PURE Sports Nutrition
  - These come in both regular and low carb options and use natural freeze dried fruits for flavour such as; Lemon, Orange, Raspberry, Superfruits and Pineapple (Low carb is only available in Lemon, Superfruits and Pineapple).
- Precision Hydration electrolytes: PH1500
  - These are the more sodium heavy, less flavour intense and a more cost friendly Hydralyte alternative. The tubes of mild citrus flavoured effervescent tablets provide a whopping 1500mg of sodium per 1L of water.
- Sodii
  - These are the perfect "purposely salty" electrolytes that combine a hit of either salty berry, salty citrus, salty pineapple or salty grapefruit flavour and oh did we mention lots of salt? These mix perfectly well in our mocktail recipes - if you're a salty sweet fan. 1 sachet provides 1000mg of sodium in just 500ml of water.

To check these brands out head to our shop (see QR code on previous page) or come in clinic and try a sample!

Recipes

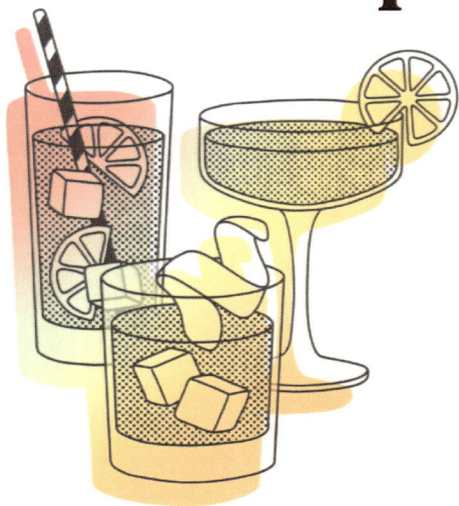

DIY Electrolytes

Ingredients (serves 4; 1 serve = 250ml)

- ¼tsp - 1 tsp salt
- 1L water
- Sweetener of choice to taste: maple syrup, honey, sugar, cordial
- Optional: any other flavouring desired. Eg: fresh fruit, lemon, lime etc

Method

1. Mix together all ingredients and enjoy!

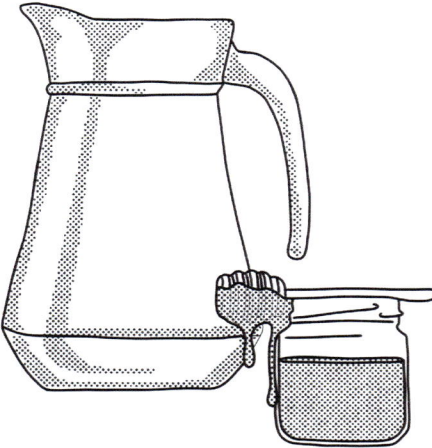

Electrolyte Mocktails

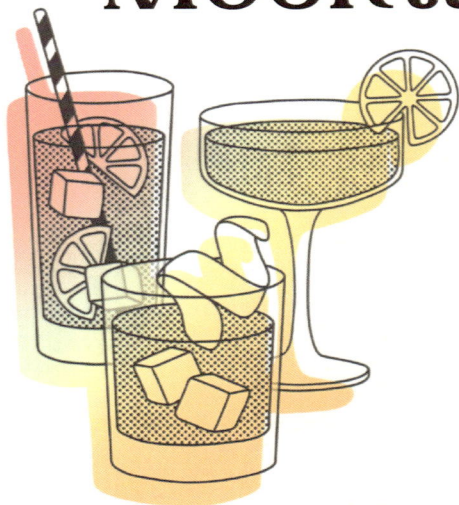

Orange Spritz

Ingredients (serves 1)

- 60 ml non-alcoholic spritz
- 90 ml non-alcoholic sparkling white wine
- 30 ml soda water
- 1 scoop PURE Sports Nutrition Orange Electrolytes
- Ice
- Garnish: sliced orange

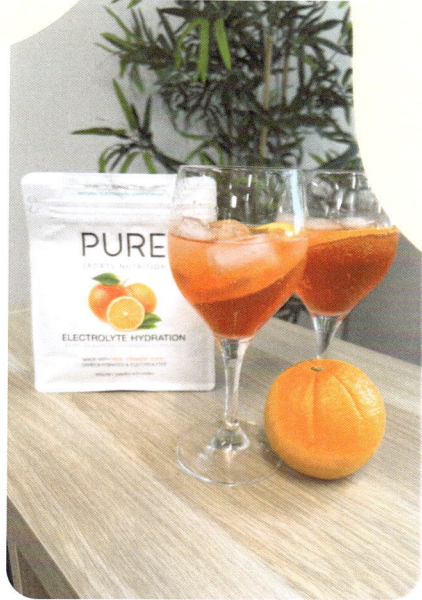

Method

1. Pour non-alcoholic spritz into a chilled wine glass.
2. Add electrolytes and stir well until dissolved.
3. Add in ice, non-alcoholic sparkling white wine, soda water, orange slice and enjoy!

Raspberry Daquiri

Ingredients (serves 1)

- 1 cup frozen raspberries
- 1/4 cup simple syrup
- 1/4 cup lime juice
- 1/4 tsp rum extract (optional)
- PURE Sports Nutrition Raspberry Electrolytes (1 scoop regular, 1/2 scoop low carb)
- Crushed Ice
- Garnish: lime wedge

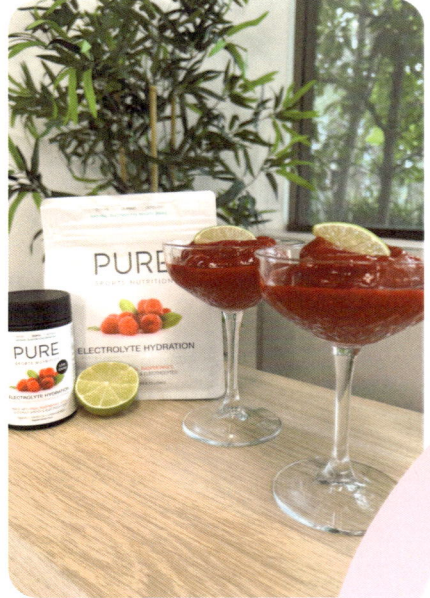

Method

1. Place all ingredients (apart from the garnish) into a blender and blend until combined.
2. Pour into a glass, garnish and enjoy!

Lemon No-Gin Fizz

Ingredients (serves 1)

- 60 ml non-alcoholic Gin (optional)
- 30 ml lemon juice
- 30 ml simple syrup
- 1/2 scoop PURE Sports Nutrition Low-Carb Lemon
- 1/2 cup soda water
- Ice
- Garnish: mint leaves and sliced lemon

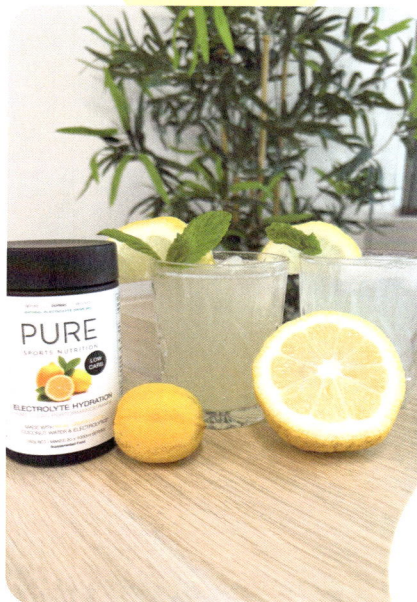

Method

1. Pour the gin, lemon juice, simple syrup and electrolytes into a cocktail shaker with ice and shake well.
2. Pour over ice into your glass, top up with soda water then garnish and enjoy!

The Sober Marg

Ingredients (serves 1)

- 1/4 cup lime juice
- 2 tbs lemon juice
- 2 tbs orange juice
- 1 tbs simple syrup or agave nectar
- 1 scoop PURE Sports Nutrition Orange or Lemon Electrolytes or 1/2 scoop PURE Sports Nutrition Lemon Low-Carb Electrolytes
- 1/4-1/2 cup soda water
- Ice
- Flaky sea salt
- Garnish: lime wedge

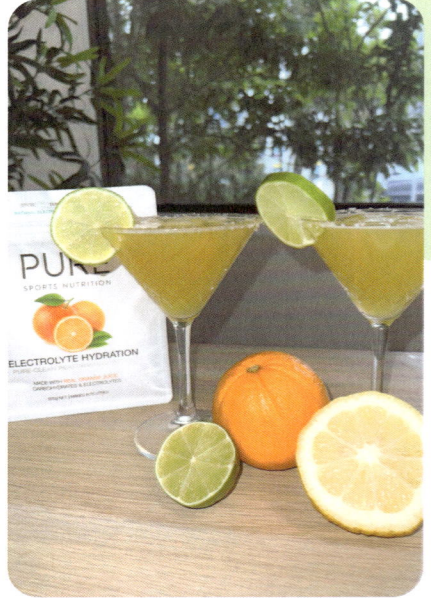

Method

1. Rim the glass with the lime wedge and sea salt.
2. Add the lime, lemon, and orange juices along with the simple syrup or agave nectar and electrolytes into a cocktail shaker and shake until mixed well.
3. Fill a glass with ice and pour over the mocktail mixture. Top up with soda water, garnish with lime and enjoy!

Grapefruit Paloma

Ingredients (serves 1)

- 60 ml grapefruit juice
- 30 ml fresh lime juice
- Sweetener of your choice, to taste (eg: sugar syrup, maple syrup, honey)
- 1/2 sachet Sodii Salty Grapefruit Electrolytes
- Sparkling water
- Ice
- Garnish: sliced grapefruit

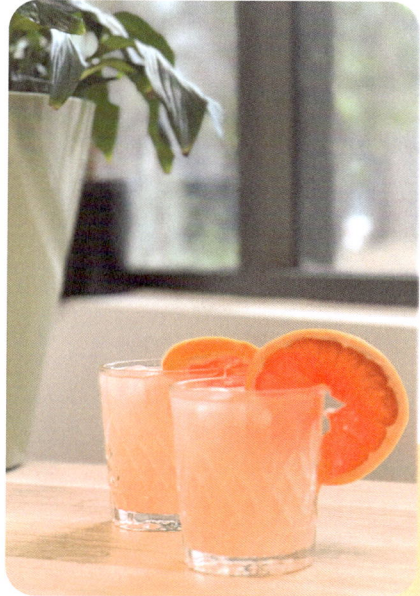

Method

1. Add the grapefruit juice, lime juice, sweetener and electrolytes to a glass and stir until well combined.
2. Fill the glass with ice.
3. Top off the glass with sparkling water, stir to combine, and serve with a slice of lime and fresh grapefruit and enjoy!

Piña Colada

Ingredients (serves 1)

- 1/4 cup coconut milk
- 1/2 cup pineapple juice
- 1 scoop PURE Sports Nutrition Pineapple Electrolytes
- 1/2 cup ice
- Garnish: fresh pineapple

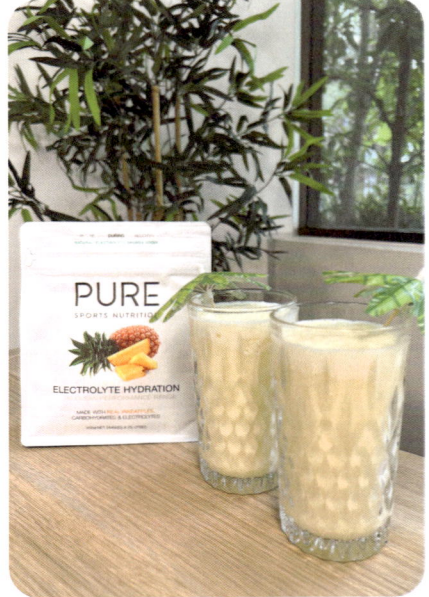

Method

1. Place all ingredients (apart from the garnish) into a blender and blend.
2. Pour into a glass and garnish with fresh pineapple and enjoy!

Matcha Mojito

Ingredients (serves 1)

- 60 ml matcha tea powder
- 150 ml Soda water (approximately)
- 1/2 scoop PURE Sports Nutrition Lemon Low-Carb Electrolytes
- 30 ml Lime or Lemon juice
- Mint
- Garnish: mint leaves and lime or lemon wedge

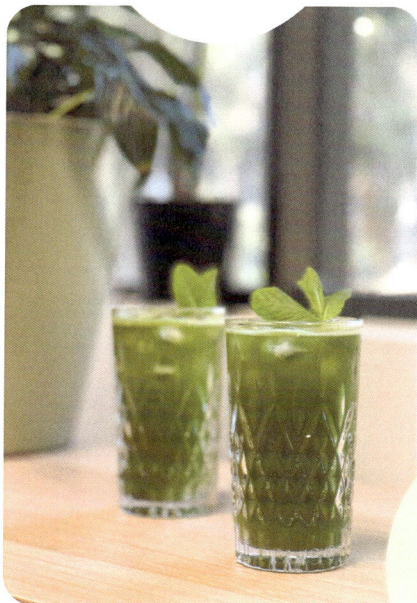

Method

1. Place some mint in the bottom of your glass and muddle to release flavour.
2. Add half of the soda water to the glass and stir in electrolytes. Be mindful to leave room in the glass as it may fizz and overflow when the electrolytes are added.
3. Top up with the rest of the soda water and stir again.
4. Add the matcha and lime/lemon juice, stir and garnish with a lime/lemon wedge, mint and serve.

Raspberry Mojito

Ingredients (serves 1)

- 1/4 cup raspberries
- 2-3 mint leaves
- Dash of lime juice
- 1/2 cup lemonade
- PURE Sports Nutrition Raspberry Electrolytes (1 scoop regular, 1/2 scoop low carb)
- Ice
- Garnish: mint leaves

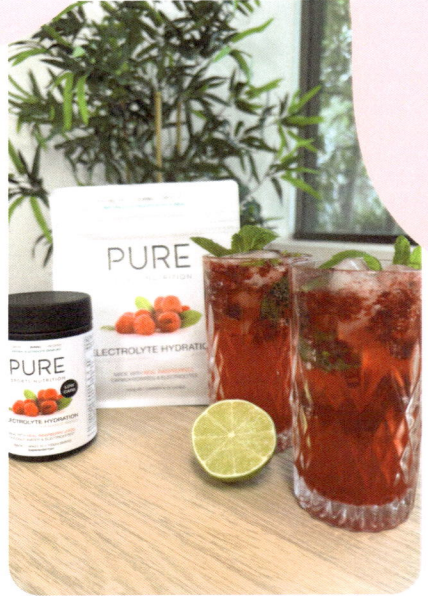

Method

1. Add the raspberries and mint to a glass and muddle until the raspberries have released their juices and the mint leaves have wilted.
2. Add the lime juice, lemonade and electrolytes and mix well then top up with ice and enjoy!

Pineapple Moscow Mule

Ingredients (serves 1)

- 60 ml pineapple juice
- 30 ml lemon juice
- 90 ml ginger beer
- 1/2 sachet Sodii Salty Pineapple Electrolytes
- Ice
- Garnishes: pineapple slice and mint

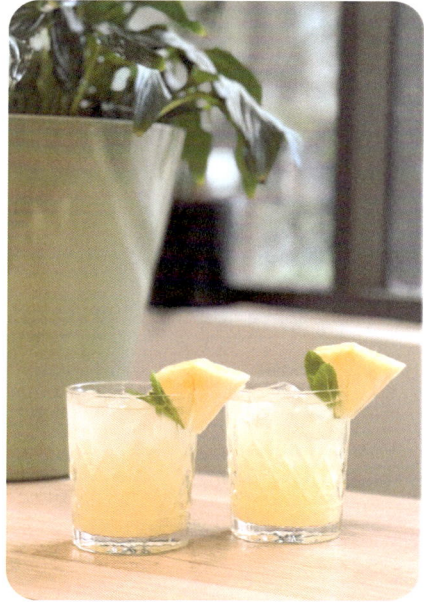

Method

1. Add the pineapple juice, lemon juice and electrolytes into a glass and stir until well combined.
2. Fill your serving glass with ice.
3. Pour the ginger beer into the serving glass.
4. Optional: add the pineapple slices and mint to the side of the glass as a garnish, and serve.

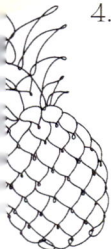

Salty Frozen Margarita

Ingredients (serves 1)

- 30 ml lime juice
- 30 ml grapefruit juice
- 30 ml orange juice
- 150 ml lime sparkling water (or plain sparkling water with lime juice)
- Sweetener of your choice, to taste (eg: sugar syrup, maple syrup, honey)
- 1/4-1/2 sachet Sodii Salty Citrus Electrolytes
- Garnish: sliced lime or lemon

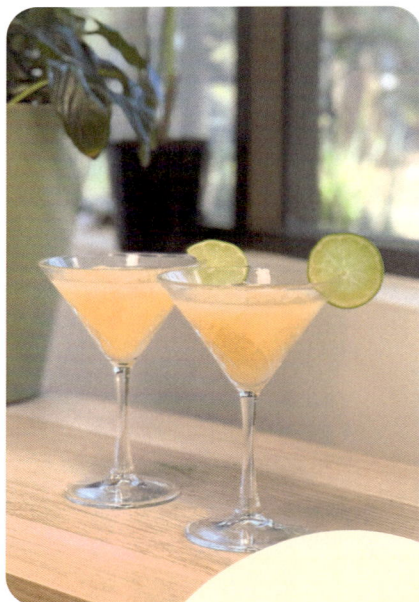

Method

1. Place juices, sweetener (if using) and electrolytes in a small jug and mix well.
2. Freeze mixture into ice cubes.
3. Place ice cubes and lime sparkling water into a blender and blend well.
4. Pour into a margarita glass and garnish with a lime wheel.

Electrolyte Jelly

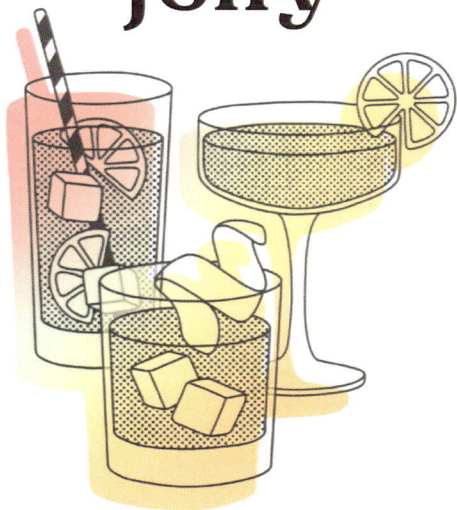

Jelly can be a fun, different and cooling way of getting in some electrolytes through a snack/dessert.

You can make either packet mix or homemade jelly with any flavour combination you would like and any electrolytes you have on hand.

We used Aeroplane Natural Colours and Flavours - Lime flavoured jelly and made half with Precision Hydration 1500 (AKA PH1500) electrolytes (mild citrus flavour) and the other half with PURE Sports Nutrition Lemon Electrolytes to create a lemon-lime electrolyte jelly!

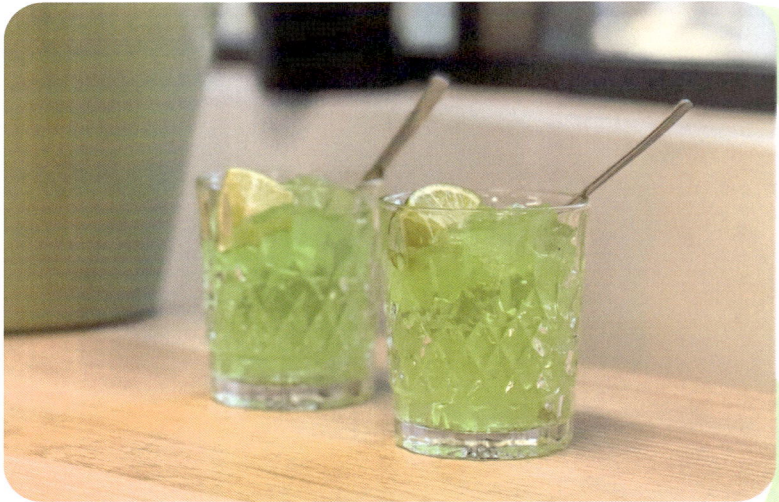

Packet Mix

Ingredients (serves 6)

- Aeroplane jelly
- Boiling water (amount directed by packet)
- Cold water (amount directed by packet)
- 0.5-1 serve of electrolytes per 250ml water used. Eg: 750ml =1.5-3 servings of electrolytes. This depends on how strong you want it/how salty your electrolytes are.
- Optional: Fruit (Do not add fresh pineapple, kiwi fruit or paw paw as jelly will not set due to their natural enzymes)

Method

1. Empty the contents of the packet into a bowl and add the boiling water. Stir and dissolve well.
2. Add electrolytes to the cold water and stir until combined or wait until dissolved. Add to the hot mixture and stir until combined.
3. Leave in a bowl or divide into glasses/jars for individual portions.
4. Add in fruit (if using).
5. Refrigerate until firm (minimum 4 hours).

Home-Made

Ingredients (serves 8)
- 4 cup juice (any juice other than pineapple)
- 2 tbs of gelatine
- 1-4 serves of electrolytes (depending on how strong you want it/how salty your electrolytes are)
- Optional: sweetener of your choice (eg: 2tbs honey, agave, sugar)

Method
1. Add 1/2-3/4 cup of the juice to a bowl or liquid measuring cup and sprinkle with gelatine powder.
2. Whisk together to combine and allow to sit for 3-5 minutes to "bloom." The granules will plump and the mixture will look like very thick applesauce or take on a lumpy appearance.
3. Pour the remaining (3 1/4- 3 1/2 cup) juice into a medium saucepan. Heat over medium heat until almost boiling.
4. Remove from heat and stir in sweetener (if using), the bloomed gelatine mixture and electrolytes. Stir to dissolve.
5. Pour into a bowl or divide into glasses/jars for individual portions.
6. Add in fruit (if using).
7. Refrigerate about 4 hours, or until set.

Electrolyte Icy Poles

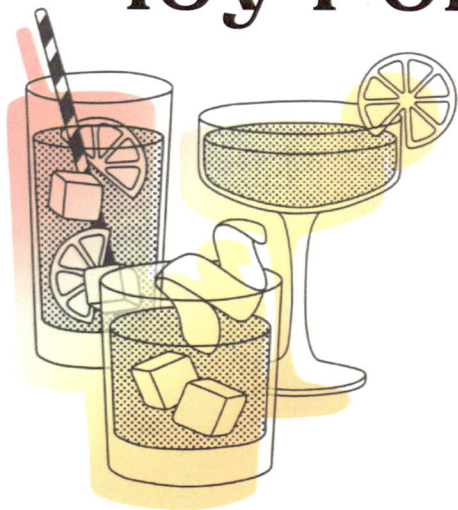

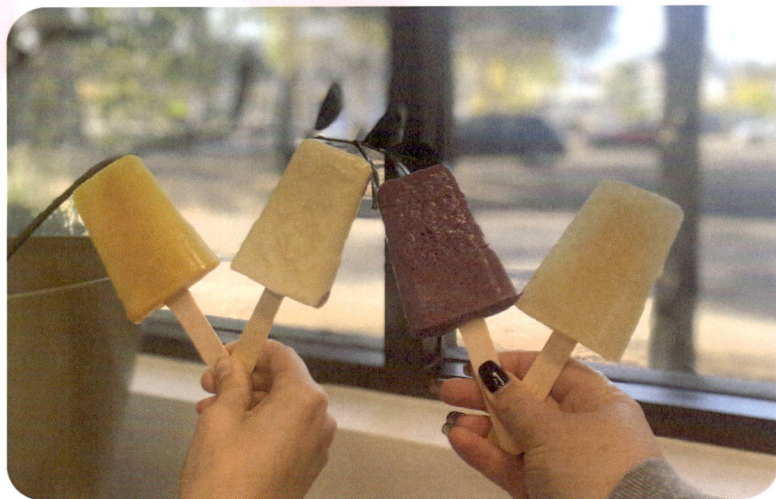

*A note on sweeteners: Sweeteners are classified as optional for these recipes (except for the Lemonade icy pole as it balances out the citrus) as it depends on the type of electrolytes you are using. We used PURE electrolytes to make these icy poles when testing and did not need to add sweetener for taste; however if using higher sodium and less sweet brands of electrolytes, we would recommend adding sweetener to taste.

Pineappsicles

Ingredients (serves 4)

- 1 1/2 cup pineapple, fresh or frozen, cut into chunks
- 1 1/4 cup Greek yoghurt or coconut cream
- 1/4 cup pineapple juice
- 1 sachet Sodii Salty Pineapple Electrolytes or 4 scoops PURE Sports Nutrition Pineapple Electrolytes
- Optional: 1 tbs sweetener*

Method

1. Combine all ingredients into a blender and process until smooth.
2. Pour into icy pole moulds, add the sticks, and freeze for a total of 8 to 12 hours until completely set.
3. To remove the icy poles, dip the moulds in warm water to loosen. Enjoy!

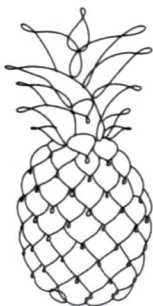

Berry Smoothie

Ingredients (serves 4)

- 1 1/2 cup Greek Yoghurt or coconut cream or 2/3 cup orange juice if you don't like your smoothies to be 'creamy'
- 1 cup fresh or frozen mixed berries
- 1-3 tbs of sweetener (honey, sugar, maple syrup etc)*
- 4 scoops PURE Sports Nutrition Electrolytes (Superfruits or Raspberry) or 1 sachet Sodii Salty Berry Electrolytes
- Optional: to make more of a satiating snack, you can add in extra fibre or other smoothie ingredients (eg: ground flaxseed or Benefiber powder for fibre, protein powder for some extra protein, nut butter for some unsaturated fats)

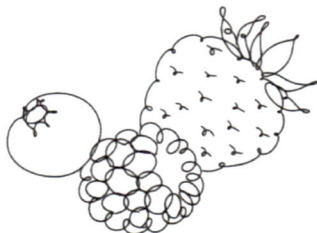

Method

1. Combine all ingredients into a blender and process until smooth.
2. Pour into icy pole moulds, add the sticks, and freeze for a total of 8 to 12 hours until completely set.
3. To remove the icy poles, dip the moulds in warm water to loosen. Enjoy!

Lemonade

Ingredients (serves 4)

- 1 1/2 cup water (1/4-1/2 cup boiled, 1-1 1/4 cold)
- 1/4-1/2 cup sweetener of your choice
- Zest from 1 lemon
- 1/2 cup lemon juice
- 4 scoops PURE Sports Nutrition Lemon Electrolytes or 1 sachet Sodii Salty Citrus Electrolytes or 1-1.5 tablet Precision Hydration - PH1500 Electrolytes

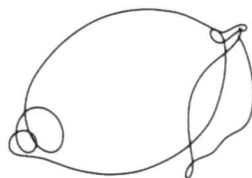

Method

1. Add equal parts boiling water and sugar into a bowl. Add in lemon zest and stir until sugar is fully dissolved.
2. In a separate bowl combine the cold water and electrolytes until dissolved.
3. Combine both hot water mixture and cold water mixture as well as the lemon juice.
4. Strain through a sieve to remove the lemon zest and any pips that have made it in. (Can skip this step if you don't mind lemon zest in your icy poles - still remove any pips).
5. Pour into icy pole moulds and freeze for 5 hours or until frozen solid. Enjoy!

Citrus Crush

Ingredients (serves 4)

- 1 1/2 cup Orange Juice
- 4 scoops PURE Sports Nutrition Orange Electrolytes or 1 sachet of Sodii Salty Citrus or Salty Grapefruit Electrolytes
- Optional: 1 tbs sweetener *

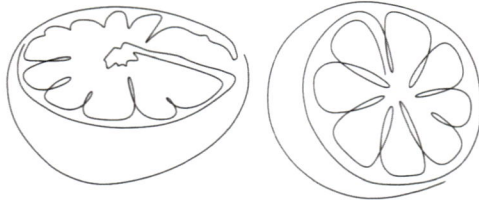

Method

1. Combine all ingredients into a jug and stir until combined and electrolytes have dissolved.
2. Pour into icy pole moulds, add the sticks, and freeze for a total of 8 to 12 hours until completely set.
3. To remove the icy poles, dip the moulds in warm water to loosen. Enjoy!

A bit about AHC ...

AHC was founded in 2008, as we noticed there was a gap in health care where such significant need of understanding and support was just missing, so we set out to focus on being just that.

As the clinic has broadened, we've expanded our knowledge, our reach and our focus and created quite a strong mission. We're aiming to make invisible illnesses, visible and we hope to do that by impacting 26 million lives by 2026, and that goal will continue to grow.

Our focus is to be a one-stop hub, a central space for those with chronic invisible illnesses to have support, understanding, safe treatment and advocacy. Knowing we have quite a mammoth journey in front of us and are hellbent on achieving it, we have our focuses to keep us true to that goal; our values.

We pride ourselves on integrity and always respecting the whole person to understand and better manage complex health conditions with access to a supportive, accepting and proactive community.

About the AHC diet team

Since 2020, our team of Dietitians have been supporting individuals with invisible illnesses, related food challenges, and gastrointestinal symptoms.

Furthermore, the Dietetics team has diligently created resources, including this recipe book, to assist and advocate for the impact invisible illnesses can have on food and nutrition. This includes discovering exciting and accessible ways to consume electrolytes to support conditions such as OI, POTS, and Dysautonomia.

We have a couple of questions for you.

Do you live with an invisible illness and experience any (or multiple) gastrointestinal symptoms including; nausea, bloating, lack of appetite, vomiting, salt cravings, reflux, early satiety (feeling of fullness), food intolerances and food reactions, food-related sensory challenges? Do you also face any other challenges related to nutrition, and food access such as; difficulties with food shopping, planning, preparing, and cooking?

If so...

You may benefit from working with an invisible illness Dietitian! You may be thinking, what is an invisible illness Dietitian and how can they help me?

Scan the below QR code for a short video on what a Dietitian can do to support those living with invisible illness.

Acknowledgements

This book was written by Mel Grande (AHC Dietitian) who also created, tested and photographed all recipes.

With many thanks to Rebecca Grande, for her beautiful and vibrant illustrations and design input which have helped the recipes shine.

Acknowledgements to the whole AHC Dietetics team; Luke Hassan, Amy Coen and Shay Poulter for their time, input and support with this book.

Further acknowledgements to the whole AHC team for arguably the best job - tasting recipes and giving honest feedback.

Lastly, we would like to thank you for your time and effort in engaging with this book and Active Health Clinic. We would like to thank you in supporting us in our mission and vision.

www.ingramcontent.com/pod-product-compliance
Lightning Source LLC
Chambersburg PA
CBRC101140030426
42334CB00008B/121